Book 1:

Essential Oils & Weight Loss for Beginners

BY LINDSEY P

&

Book 2:

Carrier Oils for Beginners

BY LINDSEY P

Book 1:

Essential Oils & Weight Loss for Beginners

BY LINDSEY P

Ultimate Guide to Losing Weight, Increasing Energy, Balancing Metabolism & Appetite Using Essential Oils & Aromatherapy

Essential Oils
&
Weight Loss
For Beginners

Ultimate Guide to Losing Weight, Increasing
Energy, Balancing Metabolism & Appetite Using
Essential Oils and Aromatherapy

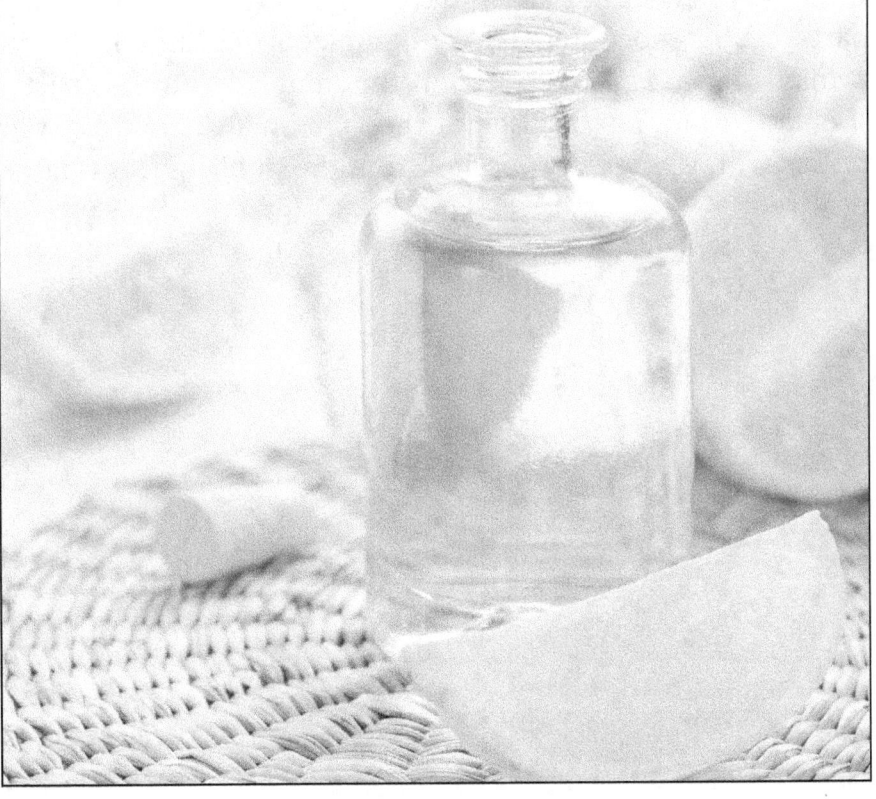

Table Of Contents

Introduction

I want to thank you and congratulate you for purchasing the book, "Essential Oils & Weight Loss for Beginners".

This book contains proven steps and strategies on how to make essentials oils work for you to help you conquer the battle against the weighing scale and measuring tape and to increase your energy and balance your metabolism.

It might sound a little far-fetched to hear that certain essential oils can actually help you to fight off your bulges. However, it is indeed possible! By the end of reading this book, you will find yourself more prepared and equipped to make essential oils work to your advantage. Read on to find out how orange peel essential oils can help turn your orange-peel skin into a cellulite-free smooth and toned skin.

Thanks again for purchasing this book, I hope you enjoy it!

Chapter 1: Essential Oils Basics

Before you get to learn which essential oils can help you in weight loss and how these can accomplish that, let us discuss first just what exactly essential oils are.

Essential oils are concentrated liquids that have a tendency to not absorb water or to not dissolve in or mix with water, it also has botanical aroma compounds that evaporate readily at normal temperature or pressure.

Oils from different kinds of plants are termed "essential" because it contains the essence or specific scent of the plant from which it was taken. It does not mean that it is essential or a must for one's health, but it sure can help us in more ways than one.

Distillation is the most common way used to extract essential oils from plants. Lavender, peppermint, and eucalyptus essential oils are the most commonly distilled oils. The different parts of the plant where the extract is to be taken from, like the roots, leaves, flowers, and others, are put inside a distillation apparatus, known as an alembic. It is then put over water and then heated. As the water's temperature rises, it will produce steam that will pass through the part of the plant, which will then vaporize the volatile elements in it. Then the vaporized compounds will then flow through a cooling coil, which will make it condense and return to a liquid state. Then the extracted liquid will then be collected in a container.

The less common processes are expression, which involves pressing the plants in a pressing device or machine to squeeze out the oils. Most citrus peels, like orange, lemon, and grapefruit, are expressed to get their essential oils. They can either be pressed mechanically or through cold-press. The peel of citrus fruits yield a large quantity of oil. In addition, growing and harvesting them takes very low cost. For this reason, essential oils from citrus fruits are less expensive compared to the cost of other essential oils.

Another way to get essential oils from plants is solvent extraction, which involves separating compounds using a funnel that separates it into two different liquids depending on their solubility. Most commonly, flowers undergo this process as they do not have enough volatile compounds for expression. Moreover, the chemical elements of flowers are too delicate and are readily denatured when heated at high temperatures using the process of steam distillation. Therefore, extraction through the use of solvents such as supercritical carbon dioxide is used to get the oils from the flowers.

Essential oils, also known as plant extracts, are used in cosmetics, soaps, perfumes, food and beverage flavoring, and other scented products. Although essential oils are not a requirement for the health, these have been applied medically throughout history as hair and skin treatments, cancer cures, aromatherapy, and others.

Western and Oriental medicine practitioners often argue about the efficacy of essential oils. Oriental or alternative medicine claims essential oils as having curative effects and many can testify to having been directly benefited by essential oils. When giving or being given acupressure or different kinds of massages, essential oils are used directly on the skin to be absorbed through the pores or diffused by nebulizers or burned as a candle or incense to be absorbed through the lungs.

If you would like to know how certain essential oils can help you to increase your metabolism, boost your energy, and help you lose weight, then please read on to the next chapter.

Chapter 2: How They Work for You

It is absolutely true that using certain essential oils can help you burn fat. However, nothing quite beats good old-fashioned proper diet and exercise. Discretion should be used when using essential oils to aid in weight loss. Never should one imagine or expect that certain essential oils are enough to keep your body fit and trimmed while you overeat and under-exercise.

That being said though, essential oils coupled with proper diet and exercise can do wonders for your body. Losing weight is not just about what you eat or what you do. It is also about how you feel about your body and about yourself.

Certain essential oils can help you when you are overeating because of certain events or experiences in your life. Let's face it. We eat our feelings every now and then. Whenever we are sorely distressed over something, we will almost instantly head to our favorite comfort food restaurant or food stall to eat a devilishly delicious and decadent chocolate cake or some hot and crispy deep fried poultry and root crops. Whichever the case, essential oils can give you comfort from whatever it is you are going through that makes you overeat with zero calories.

There are no particular essential oils that burn fat directly. However, certain essential oils can boost your metabolism, which in turn can help you in your weight loss goal and in cutting your body's fat deposits. Therefore, you must choose essential oils that aid in boosting your energy and metabolism.

Some of these energy-boosting and metabolism-balancing essential oils include citrus fruits (like oranges, lemons, bergamot, and grapefruits), herbs (like rosemary, sandalwood, and basil), and spices (like ginger, peppermint, and cinnamon).

There are many different ways in which you can mix and use these essential oils to your benefit depending on what you need them for. In the next chapter, we will talk about essential oils from citrus fruits.

Chapter 3: Citrus Essential Oils

It has long been proven by scientists that there is a strong link between what you smell, how you feel, and what eating pattern you have. Often, we take our senses for granted and do not realize just how strongly it affects our brain and behavior. You would agree that there is more than one time when your stomach grumbles like it is hungry when in fact, you just ate a short while ago and you are not actually hungry. Steadily inhaling citrus scents can help deceive our brain into thinking that our stomachs are full and therefore stopping it from sending signals to the brain that it is hungry.

The citrus family is a huge family. Citrus fruits have always benefited mankind in more ways than one. In this chapter, we will highlight the weight loss benefits of using essential oils from citrus fruits.

ORANGE. First on our list is the humble yet mighty and versatile orange. Different types of orange peels can yield their essential oils through the process of cold expression. Essential oils from different kinds of oranges are the most commonly added ingredients to various beauty products. Anti-aging creams, energizing body lotions, refreshing body wash variants, and other body care products use orange essential oils. Likewise, household items such as scented candles, aerosol deodorizing sprays for the rooms, and other scented products use orange essential oils.

Orange essential oils are also quite often used in pastries and other types of dishes as a flavoring and you would have ingested it more often than you are aware of. That being said though, you might become skeptical as to the efficacy of it since you have not felt directly any of its supposed properties in aiding you to lose weight and control your appetite.

The main reason for this is that the amount you absorb or consume is not enough for you to be able to feel the supposed effects. It can only act as a mood booster but that is pretty much the best you can get out of it. In order for you to feel the weight loss benefits, the orange essential oil must be in pure organic and undiluted form. That is why it is important to buy the pure, undiluted oils from trusted organic sources.

However, you must not confuse the fruit with the oil. The orange fruit is absolutely delicious and refreshing to the taste buds to eat. But the pure, undiluted orange oil is not to be eaten the way you would the fruit. To be able to benefit from the oil, you must use it in an aromatherapy session to help you control your cravings and cope with the everyday stress you encounter that might lead you to overeat.

You can put the orange essential oil in a diffuser to give a lingering, pleasant scent that everyone in the room can savor while the scent fills the room. If you are out and about, you can also bring a portable diffuser or inhaler so you can steadily inhale the refreshing scent of oranges for about five minutes to curb your cravings anytime you get them.

GRAPEFRUIT. The next one in line in the citrus family is the grapefruit. Grapefruit essential oils can stop your body from retaining water, which is one of the main causes of bloating, and can also dissolve fat in the body. The essential oil accomplishes this by releasing the stored fat into the bloodstream so your body can dissolve and absorb it and turn it into energy, helping you to feel energized. So you can say goodbye to your cellulites and say hello to toned thighs and arms.

Like orange essential oils, grapefruit essential oils can also be a strong suppressant for your cravings. It can help you feel fuller for longer. You can put a few drops of the grapefruit essential oil into your diffuser or inhaler to stop any hunger pangs from making you reach for another bag of chips. Another way is to put a drop of the essential oil in 8 ounces of drinking water to drink before you have your lunch or dinner. This will stop you from eating more than you should.

Grapefruit essential oils also help uplift your thoughts and moods. Improved moods can help you deal with stress better and help you have a better acceptance of yourself and your body, which can save you from developing any eating disorders, be it eating too much or too little.

You can mix different essentials oils as well to achieve better results. When you encounter extra stressful days that make you want to dive into a tub of vanilla ice cream, why not dive into your bath tub instead? Try mixing about eight drops of grapefruit essential oil and five drops of ginger essential oil to about two ounces of olive or sweet almond oil into your bath water and soak away to refreshment and relaxation.

The different essential oils you can mix together to relieve stress are lemon, chamomile, lavender, grapefruit, and jasmine essential oils. These essential oils have a calming effect. If you are depressed, uplifting and mood-boosting mixes can be of rose, sandalwood, orange, lavender, grapefruit, and jasmine essential oils. If you are feeling anxious, you can arrange for a massage and add a mixture or bergamot, sandalwood, rose, and lavender to your massage oil or as an incense to chase your anxieties away.

LEMON. Lemon essential oil is extracted from lemon rinds using cold press. It gently detoxifies the body. It relieves the body of some intestinal parasites that contribute to ill digestive health. Lemon has the ability to cleanse the body from toxins because of the antioxidant limonene. You can add a drop of lemon essential oil in a glass of water for a refreshing and uplifting drink. As with the abovementioned citrus fruits, lemon essential oil shares the same benefits for people wanting to lose weight and control their eating habits.

BERGAMOT. Bergamot is about the size of a typical orange but with a yellow rind like a lemon's. It is also used in many medicinal concoctions. Bergamot essential oils are strongly sedative and is therefore calming and best to use when you are stressed or tense that you want to reach for something decadent. So instead of letting sweets and simple sugars calm your nerves, let bergamot essential oils work for you. You will get the same calming effect without any added calories to your diet.

When paired with lavender essential oils, the calming or sedative effect will be more powerful. You can take a clean cloth and put a few drops of bergamot on it then steadily inhale it to help you relax when you are stressed out or when you get the urge to eat when you know you shouldn't. You can also dilute a drop of the oil in a teaspoon of honey and take it as you would cough syrup. Or you can make a calming yet delicious drink by diluting a drop of the oil in a small glass of almond or soy milk.

Well, now that you are acquainted with the citrus family, let us now get to know the other essential oils that will become your best friends in your war against cellulites.

Chapter 4: Non-citrus Essential Oils

In this chapter, we are going to talk about the not-so-citrus essential oils and how they can help us in expelling adipose tissues that are overstaying in our bodies.

PEPPERMINT. There is a part of your brain that tells you that your stomach is now filled with your mother's special meatloaf and that it can't accommodate anymore meatloaf. But sometimes, or should I say most of the time, we ignore what our brain tells us and listen to our eyes and taste buds telling us to eat more. Peppermint specifically works on that part of your brain to make it keep telling you that you are indeed full.

In addition, your tummy will love peppermint because it has proven itself as a great helper for digestion. It resolves a wide variety of digestive ailments. It can help you out if you are having problems with candida, as it is often a big influence in your losing or gaining weight. Moreover, when you are under heavy emotions like depression or anxiety, it can uplift and lighten your mood and motivate you to be more optimistic. And most importantly, peppermint tastes amazing and will let you give a minty fresh kiss to your special someone as well.

Before you eat anything, put a couple of drops of peppermint essential oil to a clean cloth or a cotton pad and steadily breathe in vapors. You can also put the drops in a diffuser and inhale your way to a reduced appetite. Likewise, you can put a drop of the peppermint oil in a glass of water for a refreshing drink before each meal. You can also pair it with lemon to get the most energizing and waistline-reducing effect.

SANDALWOOD. Sandalwood essential oils also have calming sedative properties that can help you control your eating habits when you are undergoing stressful situations. Sandalwood helps you combat negative feelings and actions. The feeling of having conquered negativity with relieve you of the stress you were having and so relieving you as well of the impulse to eat something comforting like you beloved mother's macaroni and cheese.

Sandalwood essential oils may be used with a diffuser and constantly inhaling the vapors. You can also dilute a drop of the sandalwood oil in a drop of extra virgin olive oil and then apply it directly on your feet or stomach for faster absorption. You can also take it like you would any medical syrup by adding a drop of sandalwood essential oil to a teaspoon of honey. You can also make a delicious drink by mixing a drop of the sandalwood oil to a small glass of rice milk.

GINGER. The lowly ginger is quite famous in Asian cuisine for being tummy-friendly. It is this spicy yet mildly sweet ingredient that makes Asian dishes taste really good. But its being tummy-friendly is not just because it makes dishes taste awesome. It is also loved by your stomach because of its anti-inflammatory and anti-bacterial properties that makes the stomach healthy and in tip-top shape.

In addition, ginger also has a warming effect on the body because of its being mildly spicy, stimulating the body, especially the nervous system. Ginger essential oil has been dubbed as the "oil of empowerment" as it gives off a mild heat that stimulates our inner strength, energizing and empowering the body and the mind.

To get the full benefit of ginger essential oil, you can put a couple of drops in a diffuser and inhale the vapors as you would any other essential oils that we have already discussed. You can also apply it directly to your skin or by diluting it first in coconut oil if you have sensitive skin. You can do a skin test first by applying it to your forearm to see if you are sensitive to it or not.

CINNAMON. Cinnamon is known to increase the weight loss effectiveness of all the other essential oils you have read about in this book. Diabetics can find comfort in knowing that cinnamon has been discovered to trigger healthy levels of insulin in the body. It also improves digestion and blood circulation. Its antioxidant properties help in gently detoxifying the body and stimulating the immune system to get to fight against invaders that try to give us colds and flu.

Cinnamon essential oil taken from the cinnamon leaves and twigs through steam distillation has a mildly spicy and musky scent. Cinnamon is great in aromatherapy. However, cinnamon oil from the cinnamon bark in not usually used in aromatherapy. Much like ginger essential oils, cinnamon essential oils are also mildly spicy and so it warms up the body as well and fights against exhaustion and depression by empowering the body.

In aromatherapy, you can put a few drops of the cinnamon essential oil in burners or vaporizers to be inhaled steadily to calm you and take your mind off eating out of stress. You can also dilute the oil in your bath water as you soak all your worries away. In addition, you can also simultaneously fight off any outwardly infections while soaking in your cinnamon infused bath water because of the cinnamon oil's antiseptic properties.

Chapter 5: A Helper and Complement

These essential oils that we have discussed in this book will only be effective if you work hard at your goal as well. Remember that nothing can replace proper diet and regular exercise to help you keep fit and healthy. But these essential oils can greatly help you in your struggle against whether to pick up that mouth-watering sandwich and take a bite off of it when you are not genuinely hungry.

These previously mentioned essential oils will boost you the two other main weapons in your war against excess fat. These essential oils have different properties that work to help you in breaking down fat in order to be fully absorbed by your body and turned into energy. They help curb your appetite and your "midnight-snack" cravings. They affect the part of the brain to help you relax and calm down instead of converting your anxieties and stresses into overeating.

Of course, disciplining yourself to eat the right kinds of food and to have a regular exercise program is difficult at first. You might be dreading or avoiding having to eat healthy food or having to go to the gym or just increase your daily physical activity. It might be the very reason that you have bought this book trying to find a way to lose weight without having to follow a proper diet and a regular exercise plan.

Well, following the instructions above and using essential oils alone in your goal of losing weight is indeed a possibility. It is not impossible. However, it is not enough and all the more so if you continue to live a sedentary lifestyle and choose unhealthy kinds of food. There should be balance in everything. One way or another, you are going to have to face the consequences of your actions (or for that matter, lack of action).

It is not at all daunting to follow a proper diet plan and a regular exercise program. But first, you have to want to make yourself healthier. Without your will and motivation, you most probably will not succeed. Moreover, you need to be consistent and steady with your routine to reach your goal of losing weight and keeping fit. If you are not consistent, you will undergo a yo-yo pattern, in which you will lose weight when you are motivated and gain weight when you are not.

It is not only bad for your health, it is also bad for your physical appearance as well because a yo-yo diet will ruin the elasticity of your skin causing it to have stretch marks and that will not be a very nice sight to see. Losing weight gradually coupled with good exercise will give your skin time to adjust to fit your new size, reducing the possibility of stretch marks and skin flaps that are commonly seen in people undergoing crash diets.

The food you eat also plays a big role in your goal to losing weight. Aside from keeping your body healthy in general, vitamins in fruits and vegetables, particularly vitamins A and E, will greatly increase your skins elasticity and give you a rosy glow on your cheeks suggesting you are indeed in the "pink of health".

The essential oils discussed in this book will be your ally in keeping a regular exercise routine. Orange and peppermint essential oils will perk you up and keep you feeling energized and motivated to follow your exercise program. Cinnamon and ginger essential oils will empower you to keep going even when you feel like you can't go on anymore.

Sandalwood and bergamot essential oils will calm and relax your nerves when you are feeling stressed out so you can win against the temptations of rich desserts and deep fried foods. And the best part about these essential oils is that it gives no side effects as it is pure and having no caffeine, no sugar, no preservatives.

A word of caution though. You may find some shops selling essential oils, usually containing a mixture of grapefruit, coconut, cedar, and other essential oils, claiming to burn fat. It would be great for calming and energizing you as discussed above. However, these cannot really help you to break down fat or cellulite in your body. It may temporarily make your skin look firmer because it hydrates your skin, but it is not a permanent fix.

It is better to research and experiment about which aromatherapy works best for you. Make sure that you do your homework and that you know how to properly use diffusers or inhalers to get the best out of your essential oils. When applying the essential oils directly on your body, make sure you dilute it first in a carrier oil such as virgin olive oil or coconut oil. Remember as well that some essential oils can be toxic to you if you directly ingest it. Always keep them in a safe place away from young children. Unless you have been using the essential oils for some time, only follow specific recipes to make sure it is safe for you.

Chapter 6: A Look in the Mirror

A mirror helps you to see yourself to check if you need to adjust your tie, if you need to reapply your lipstick, or if you have a piece of red bell pepper stuck to your teeth. But sometimes people forget to look at their inner mirror to check if the way they think or see things is correct. You need to take a good long look at yourself as well.

You need to honestly ask yourself whether you are doing this for yourself, to make yourself a better and healthier person or whether you are doing this just to please someone else. It is true that you need to present yourself well and make sure you look presentable when dealing with other people. But you should not change yourself just to please someone who does not genuinely care about you.

The motivation to lose weight should come from you, not from somebody else. Moreover, you should do it for the right reasons. When you are guided by a proper motivation and you have the right reasons to embark on the journey to weight loss, you will have more stability and consistency all throughout.

You will have a reason to go on even when you encounter setbacks in your goals, such as an unexpected dinner celebration for your friend's promotion or a relapse into pigging out during a family reunion, which ruins your carefully planned out diet, or a surprise added workload, which meant you would have to give up going to the gym for a few days to accommodate the added workload.

You need to be able to motivate yourself to continue even when setbacks happen. However, you will not always be strong. Therefore, having a loved one or a friend know of your goals and asking for their support will greatly help you win the war against your bulges. You can also have a "weight loss buddy" whom you can be with as you journey towards a better health and a better self.

Having someone to exercise and eat proper amounts and right kinds of food with will make exercising and dieting less boring and tiresome. Knowing that you are in this together will empower you more while you let the essential oils work their magic to boost your energy. You can take essential oil-infused baths together or have your massages using your favorite essential oils together.

Not only will you be benefited by your regular exercise program, your proper healthy diet, and the essential oils we have discussed in this book, but you will also be benefited by the soothing and calming effect of human connection. All these things add up to make your whole weight loss journey more pleasant. Remember that those are puzzle pieces that need to be put together in order for you to complete the picture.

Conclusion

Thank you again for purchasing this book!

I hope this book was able to help you to realize the hidden potential of certain essential oils in weight loss, in increasing your body's energy, in uplifting your mood and countenance, and in improving your overall well-being.

The next step is to apply what you have learned in this book and to get you going on your way to physical fitness and better health. Remember that these facts about the essential oils mentioned above will be useless if you do not work hard and work steady. Avoid the yo-yo and crash diets. Slow and steady wins the race too. And in the race to weight loss, the fast and furious method won't really cut it. Take your time and enjoy your journey to a thinner and more healthy you!

Finally, if you enjoyed this book, please take the time to share your thoughts and post a review on Amazon. We do our best to reach out to readers and provide the best value we can. Your positive review will help us achieve that. It'd be greatly appreciated!

Thank you and good luck!

Book 2:

Carrier Oils for Beginners

BY LINDSEY P

Discover the Characteristics and Beauty and Health Benefits of Carrier Oils for mixing Aromatherapy Essential Oils

CARRIER OILS
FOR
BEGINNERS

Discover The Characteristics, beauty and
health benefits of carrier oils for mixing
Aromatherapy Essential Oils

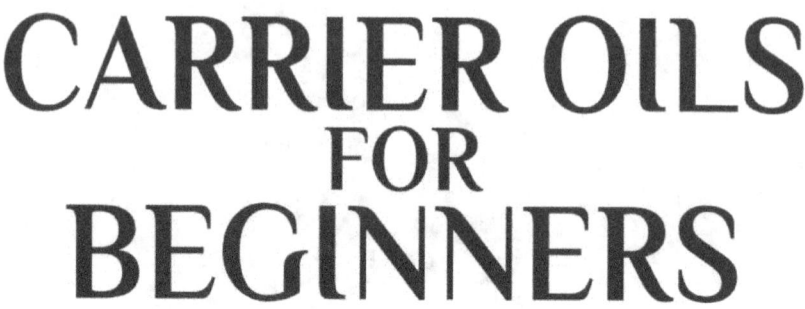

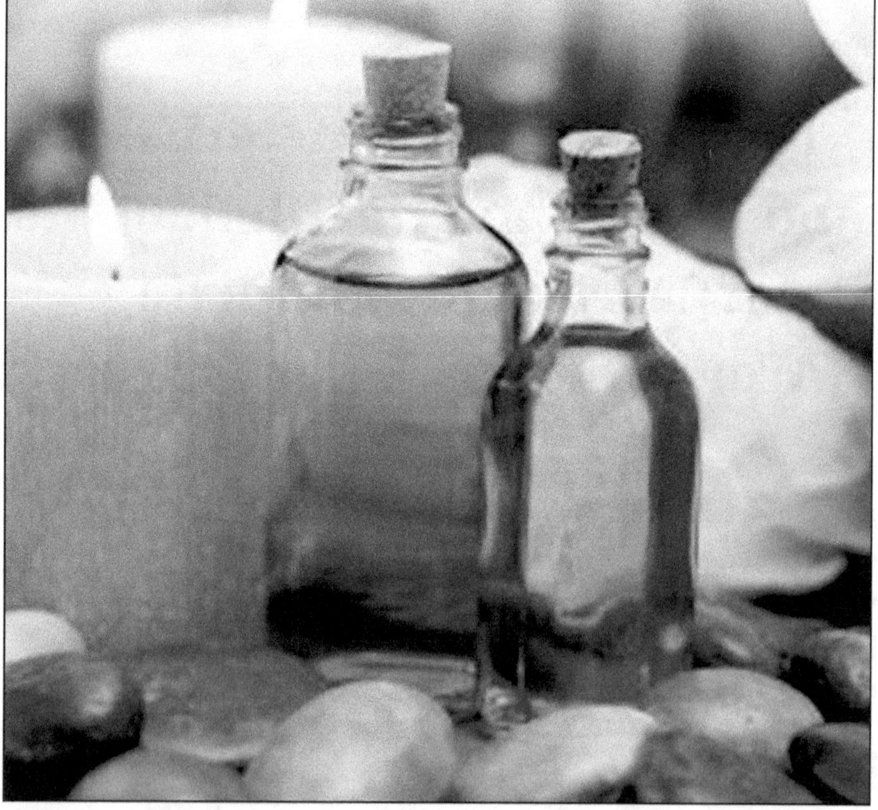

Table of Contents

Introduction

I want to thank you and congratulate you for purchasing the book, *"Carrier Oils for Beginners: Discover the Characteristics and Beauty and Health Benefits of Carrier Oils for Mixing Aromatherapy Essential Oils."*

This book discusses what carrier oils really are and what the different types of this oil are. This book also talks about the benefits of carrier oils (both for health and beauty). And lastly, this book contains proven steps and strategies on how to mix carrier oils with aromatherapy essential oils to enjoy its maximum benefits.

If you like to know more about carrier oil and what it can do for you, then this book is definitely for you!

Thanks again for purchasing this book, I hope you enjoy it!

Chapter 1: An Introduction to Carrier Oils

Carrier oils, which are also called as base oils, are types of oils that are being used to dilute another type of oil that is called the essential oil. It is important to mix carrier oils with essential oils because the latter can be too concentrated when applied to skin undiluted. Therefore, before you can even use essential oils for aromatherapy and massage, you first have to dilute them by adding the carrier oils.

More so, carrier oils are called as such because they "carry" the essential oils onto a person's skin, especially during aromatherapy. They make it easier for the skin as well as the blood system of a person to absorb the oil easier and better.

Carrier oils are one of those organic and natural oils that do not have scents or any concentrated aroma (although there are few that have distinct mild smell, such as the olive oils). This type of oil also does not evaporate because they are not as volatile as the essential oils.

In using carrier oils, people usually make sure that these oils are as natural and as pure as it can possibly be because they believe that organic oils are of much higher quality and work so much better than those that are adulterated already.

Carrier oils also require a specific method of growing since they have to be as pure as possible. This is most applicable when you are going to use carrier oils for therapeutic purposes. You have to make sure that the carrier oils that you use are organically grown—not artificially grown wherein chemicals have already been applied—and cold pressed. Always remember that carrier oils are being mixed with essential oils for aromatherapy (which of course involves the human skin) so they are going to be absorbed by the human body. Therefore, it is important that the oils you use are organic and pure so that there will not be any unwanted substances that will be absorbed by the skin along with these oils.

Generally, carrier oils are important since they serve us with a wide array of benefits, not just for our health but also for our beauty (These two, of course, also intersects with each other). Carrier oils not just help the skin absorb the essential oils better; they also help the skin get moisturized. Carrier oils also protect the skin from any damage that external factors can bring. (More benefits of carrier oils will be discussed in the next chapter of this book.)

There are different types of carrier oils that are used for different purposes. Each variety of carrier oils has its own characteristics and purposes. (This will be further discussed in the third chapter of this book.) This will show you that carrier oils are indeed wonderful and important to us.

Chapter 2: Benefits of Carrier Oils

Since most of the time carrier oils serve as an aid for diluting essential oils, people usually think that carrier oils are not that important. They often times regard carrier oils as less important than essential oils and take the former for granted. However, you should realize that carrier oils must not be thought of that way. Carrier oils are as important as any other oils out there.

Carrier oils serve us really well. Contrary to what most people think, carrier oils are of much higher importance than any other things when it comes to aromatherapy. As a matter of fact, according to the Isis Essentials Carrier Oil Guide, the treatment being used in aromatherapy consists of around 98 percent carrier oils, and just about 2 percent essential oil. Carrier oils carry essential oils onto our skin during aromatherapy, so majority of the treatment consistency has to be carrier oils.

Aside from aromatherapy, carrier oils are also being used in some facial treatments, and most of these treatments consist mainly of carrier oils as well. The Isis Essentials Carrier Oil Guide also said that 99 percent of the facial treatments that are usually used nowadays are carrier oils, and only 1 percent is essential oils.

Carrier oils, when perfectly combined with essential oils, can work like charm for our skin. This mixture can make your skin softer and can even remove some wrinkles. This treatment can also bring flexibility as well as radiance to the human skin.

CARRIER OILS FOR BEGINNERS

Carrier oils are indeed as important as essential oils or any other oils.

Chapter 3: Varieties of Carrier Oils

Each kind of carrier oils has its own characteristics that make it distinct from the others. Generally, carrier oils are beneficial to our skin as well as to our health. But specifically, each type of carrier oils has its own roles and brings us different benefits.

In this chapter, we will talk about ten common carrier oils that can easily be found and are available practically anywhere.

Grape seed Oil

Grape seed oil (scientific name: *Vitus vinifera*) is a type of carrier oils that comes out of seed of grapes. This oil is being extracted whenever grape seeds are being pressed, which makes it a common by-product of the process of winemaking. However, there are only some specific varieties of grapes—reisling grapes, of example—that are used for the extraction of grape seed oil. The process of oil extraction is also quite complex, so it is important that you are aware of the method of extraction of the oil that you are going to buy.

According to the book *Carrier Oils for Aromatherapy and Massage* by Len Price, the consistency of grape seed oils usually contains about 69 percent linoleic acid (which is an essential omega-6 fatty acid), 15 percent oleic acid (an omega-9 fatty acid), 11 percent saturated fat, and less than 1 percent alpha linolenic acid (an essential omega-3 fatty acid).

The appearance of grape seed oil is usually clear, with slight and unnoticeable hint of yellow or green color. It usually smells slightly sweet and nutty and its viscosity is thin. Grape seed oils usually last for six months to a year.

Grape seed oils are also helpful in treating acnes. They have anti-inflammatory properties as well as antioxidants, which are best used for treating acnes. Since grape seed oils consist mainly of linoleic acid, they can also be used for boosting the health of your skin and preventing the occurrences of acne. Moreover, grape seed oils help close up the pores of your skin, which in turn prevents clogging and oiliness, which are common causes of acnes.

Aside from the benefits to our skin, grape seed oils can also be used in cooking. Since this oil has a relatively high smoking point, there are some people that use this oil when frying. Some also use grape seed oils for dressings and sauces.

Sweet Almond Oil

Another variety of carrier oils is the sweet almond oil (scientific name: *Prunus amygdalus var. dulcus*). This oil is considered as an "affordable all-purpose" carrier oil, which means it is practical and important to keep this oil on hand.

Price also mentioned the consistency of this oil: which is approximately 65 percent oleic acid, 27 percent linoleic acid, and 8 percent saturated fat.

Sweet almond oil usually appears clear with a bit of yellowing hint. The viscosity of this oil is medium and it smells somewhat sweet and nutty. If you store this all-around oil, it will usually last for a year.

Of course, sweet almond oil has its own share of benefits as well. Basically, this oil makes our skin healthier, since it is rich in Vitamins A, B, and E. These vitamins are known to be helpful for keeping our skin in good condition—which is why most skin care products contain these vitamins). Almond oils also maintain the level of moisture in our skin by quickly penetrating our skin without clogging the pores.

Almonds also remove all the impurities on our skin and even eliminate the dead skin cells. The dull appearance of our skin is caused by several impurities such as pollution and dirt. Sweet almond oil protects our skin from all these impurities. Moreover, this oil also gets rid of any dead skin cells, which in turn makes our skin glow brighter.

This oil is not just beneficial to our skin, but to our hair as well. In fact, sweet almond oil helps our hair stay long and healthy, since it is a rich source of magnesium. Magnesium is helpful in preventing hair fall, which is why most hair products have magnesium. Almond oil also helps us get rid of split ends (you have to apply the oil onto your hair once or twice a week) as well as dandruff (since it works by removing dead skin cells).

Sweet almond oil also helps boosting our memory since it is rich in omega-3 fatty acids as well as mono-saturated fats. Almond oil helps boost our nervous and immune systems as well.

Olive Oil

Olive oil (scientific name: *Olea europaea*) is also another type of carrier oil that are being widely used nowadays.

According to Price, olive oils consist of 60 percent oleic acid, 11 percent linoleic acid, 10 percent saturated fat, and less than one percent alpha linoleic acid.

The color of olive oils is light to medium green. The smell of this oil is also reminiscent of the Virgin Coconut Oil and the shelf like lasts for a year or two. And because this oil is very thick and its texture is very oily, there are some people who would rather use other oils that this one, especially for aromatherapy and skin care treatments.

In using olive oil, you have to make sure that you mix the right amount of this oil with other oil—especially in diluting essential oil—this may overpower the blend. Moreover, when you are to use olive oil, make sure that you use the cold-pressed and unadulterated oil.

Olive oil is also known for its health benefits. In fact, some experts suggest an intake of at least two tablespoons of virgin olive oil every day since it is good for our health.

One major benefit that olive oils give to us is its ability to protect us from heart disease. Essentially, olive oil works in the reduction of blood cholesterol levels. High level of blood cholesterol will in turn lead to heart disease.

It is also said that olive oil helps in keeping our heart healthy. We all know that as we grow older, our heart also does. There can be possible ailments in our system, such as malfunctioning of the arteries, due to aging. Therefore, it will be helpful if we take diet rich in olive oil since—according to studies—it can help improve the arterial functioning of our system as we grow older.

Avocado Oil

Avocado oil (scientific name: *Parsea americana*) is also a known variety of carrier oils. Avocado is very popular since it can easily be found. This oil is just extracted mainly from the flesh of an avocado fruit. The process of extracting the oil from the avocado is done through cold pressing.

Price also estimated the composition of avocado oils: 66 percent oleic acid, 19 percent saturated fat, 12 percent linoleic acid, and less than 5 percent alpha linoleic acid. More so, Price also suggests that avocado oils must not be put inside the refrigerator because there is a possibility that some fragile components of this oil will be affected.

As to its appearance, avocado oils look somewhat deep olive green in color. It is also highly viscous. It smells fatty, sweet, and nutty as well. Usually, avocado oils can last up to one year.

Avocado oils are a great help when it comes to taking care of our skin. This oil is rich in vitamin E, which is essential in making our dry skin rejuvenated. As a matter of fact, vitamin E is one of the most commonly used substances when it comes to skin care products. Avocado oil is also safe for the skin, so you can apply it daily. You can even add other oils (e.g. lavender oil) to this oil, yet the chemical structure will not be affected.

You can also use avocado oils to moisturize your skin, since it contains the substance called humectants (specifically, the avocado's peel contain this substance). It is suggested that you do this application during the night—just before you go to bed—and leave it on your face overnight.

When you wake up the next morning, you should then wash the oil off your face.

Avocado oil can also help in treating dry scalp. More so, avocado oil will work best if you blend it with castor oil. Just mix 2 tablespoons of avocado oil with the same amount of castor oil. Afterwards, you have to warm the mixture up before you apply it right before you go to bed. Just make sure that you rinse the oil off your head with shampoo the very next morning.

Lastly, avocado oil is also known to be effective when it comes to reducing skin aging signs. Since this oil is rich in vitamin E, it can act as an antioxidant, which in turn will fight the free radicals.

Peanut oil

Peanut oil (scientific name: *Arachis hypogeae*) is also another variety of carrier oils, which is clearly extracted from peanuts. It is also one of the common carrier oils since peanuts can be easily found.

Price said that the estimated composition of peanut oils is as follows: 50 percent oleic acid, 25 percent linoleic acid, 17 percent saturated fat, and less than one percent alpha linoleic acid.

Peanut oils appear to be virtually clear, and its viscosity is thick. They smell light with hint of fatty and nutty smell. And just like some of the other carrier oils, peanut oils also last for a year.

This type of carrier oils is used in different ways. One benefit that peanut oils can give us is that it can help energize our body. Just massage this oil onto your body, and you will eventually feel energized. More than that, massaging your body using peanut oil can also help you get rid of aching muscles as well as joints.

Moreover, peanut oils aids in the prevention of coronary artery disease and other heart problems. Although peanuts have high calorie content, it is rich in mono-saturated fatty acid (MUFA), which decreases the so-called bad cholesterol. In turn, MUFA increases the good cholesterol in our blood.

Aside from these, peanut oils can also be a great help in eliminating acnes. Just apply a few drops of this oil and then combine it with around two to three drops of lime juice. Afterwards, just apply the mixture onto the part of your skin that is infected by acnes.

However, you have to be aware that peanut oil is still made up of substances the same as peanuts (since it is from peanuts). So if you are allergic to peanuts, then you are not in any way allowed to use peanut oils.

Pecan Oil

Another variety of carrier oils is the pecan oil (scientific name: *Carya pecan*), which are extracted from pecan nuts.

Pecan oils consist approximately of 52 percent oleic acid, 36 percent linoleic acid, 7 percent palmitic, 2 percent stearic, and 1 percent linoleic acid.

Pecan oils usually appear virtually clear and it has a medium viscosity. It has a very light nutty aroma and it usually lasts for about a year.

This variety of carrier oil is known to have high fiber content, which in turn helps in boosting our cardiovascular health. Pecan oils are important in minimizing the possibility of having coronary heart disease as well as some types of cancer. Moreover, pecan oils have monosaturated fats—such as the oleic acid—as well as the phenolic antioxidants, which are both healthy for our heart.

More so, pecan oils are also helpful when it comes to the health of our digestive system. The fiber contents of pecans are essential in improving the health of our colon as well as in aiding bowel movements regularly.

There are also some researches that prove how pecan oil can be helpful in losing weight. It has been shown that having foods that contain nuts such as pecan can help you lose weight since it boosts satiety as well as metabolism.

Pecans also have anti-inflammatory advantages. They are known to be rich in magnesium that in turn eliminates inflammatory indicators in our body. An example of these inflammatory indicators is the C-reactive protein (CRP). Moreover, it lessens the possibility of having some inflammatory diseases such as cardiovascular disease, Alzheimer's disease, and arthritis.

Sesame Seed Oil

Sesame seed oil (scientific name: *Sesamum indicum*) is a type of carrier oil that is ideal to use for massage. It is also said that this oil works better is mixed with other types of carrier oil.

Sesame seed oil is composed primarily of 44 percent linoleic acid, 40 percent oleic acid, 16 percent unsaturated fat, and less than one percent alpha linoleic acid.

This type of carrier oil is a bit yellowish in color, but somewhat pale, and its viscosity ranges between medium and thick viscosity. It also smells like nutty sesame and the aroma is distinctively sweet. It also lasts for about a year.

You may opt to use this oil for hair care as well. Applying and massaging this oil onto your scalp helps make your hair color darker. It even helps in reducing hair fall. Moreover, sesame oil also helps eliminate as well as prevent dandruff, since it kills the bacteria that bring about hair and scalp problems.

Aside from the hair, our skin also benefits from sesame seed oil. As a matter of fact, this oil can act as skin moisturizer as well as soothing and anti-inflammatory remedy, which make our skin healthier. It can also block some toxins and bacteria from entering your skin and then wash these unwanted substances away.

Sesame oil also brings about healthy bones since it contains essential nutrients that are good for the bones. Sesame seed oil contains mineral zinc, which generally makes our bones healthy. This oil also has copper that aids in relieving rheumatoid arthritis. It also has some calcium mineral which in turn prevents the possibility of having osteoporosis as well as colon cancer.

Hazelnut Oil

Another variety of carrier oils is the hazelnut oil (scientific name: *Corylus avellana*). This oil is extracted from cold pressed as well as roasted hazelnuts.

Hazelnut oils are composed of 74 percent oleic acid, 17 percent linoleic acid, 9 percent saturated fat, and less than 1 percent alpha linoleic acid.

These hazelnut oils usually appear yellowish (light) and it smells somewhat lightly sweet and nutty. The viscosity of this oil is thin. Moreover, this oil usually lasts for a year, just like most carrier oils.

Generally, hazelnuts are well-known as a good source of vitamin E, an essential vitamin for keeping our heart other body muscles healthy. Vitamin E is also a good aid in eliminating some free radicals off our skins.

Hazelnut oils also play an important role in moisturizing our skin, since it contains a good amount of essential fatty acids (e.g. linoleic acid). So if you want to prevent your skin from drying—and rather rehydrate it—it will a lot helpful if you are going to apply hazelnut oil onto your skin. Hazelnut oils also do not bring about any side effects unlike some skin care products, so it is totally safe to use them even daily.

In aromatherapy, hazelnut oil also bring about a soothing feeling whenever your body is being massaged using this oil. It helps relieve physical—and even mental—stresses as your body starts to relax. Of course, the massage itself helps you relax, but it will be better if hazelnut oil is used since it regenerates your cells as well as strengthens all your capillaries.

If you do not have sunscreen to use, then hazelnut oil can also be a good alternative. This oil can help protect your skin from excessive exposure to harmful sun rays. In fact, most sunscreens have hazelnut contents. It is also suggested that you mix hazelnut oil with other carrier oils (e.g. avocado oil and sesame oil) for better results. You can also add a drop of hazelnut oil to your lotion and cream so that, when applied, it can act as a guard for your skin.

Sunflower Oil

Sunflower oil (scientific name: *Helianthus annuus*) is also a type of carrier oil that can be easily found anywhere, since sunflower is not a rare type of flower. More than that, sunflower oils are also affordable in the market, and they can be used in any purpose.

Generally, sunflower oil has the following components: 64 percent linoleic acid, and about 12 percent saturated fat. Standard sunflower oils usually have around 20 percent oleic acid, which High Oleic sunflower oils have around 80 percent oleic oil (which is why they are called High Oleic).

The color of this oil is virtually clear, though there is a light hint of yellow. It also has thin viscosity and it smells sweet and faint. Just like most carrier oils, sunflower oil usually lasts for about a year.

Sunflower oil helps in fighting free radicals since—just like most carrier oils—it also has high level of vitamin E. It is also rich in tocopherols, which are essential in fighting free radicals that cause cancer.

This variety of carrier oil also helps prevent arthritis as well as asthma. Therefore, it will be helpful if you include sunflower oil to your diet. You may use this oil for frying as well as for dressing.

Watermelon Seed Oil

Watermelon seed oil (scientific name: *Citrullus vulgaris*) is also a type of carrier oil that is beneficial to us. Of course, this oil is extracted from the seeds of the watermelon fruit.

This carrier oil is yellow in color and it smells somehow nutty. It is also lightly viscous. And unlike most carrier oils, watermelon seed oil lasts for quite a very long time, since it is highly stable and its shelf life is indefinite.

Watermelon seeds, in general, are a good source of important minerals and nutrients. Of course, watermelon seed oil also contains these important elements, so it is indeed essential to our health.

Watermelon seeds contain magnesium, which is important in keeping the normal functioning of our heart as well as normal blood pressure. Magnesium also helps in facilitating our body's metabolism and even protein synthesis.

Moreover, the seeds of a watermelon fruit are also rich in lycopene. As we all know, lycopene is a strong antioxidant that is important in preventing our cells from getting damaged. Likewise, lycopene are also good in keeping our face healthy.

Chapter 4: Mixing Carrier Oils with Essential Oils for Aromatherapy

As mentioned in Chapter 1, carrier oils are mainly used to dilute essential oils, since the latter can't be applied onto the human skin undiluted. Due to its high concentration, essential oils should be mixed with carrier oils to that it can be safely used.

Diluting essential oils with carrier oils should be taken seriously. Everything should be handled with care. You must choose which type of carrier oil is perfect to use. Of course, you have to use the oil which has a high quality—it is even preferable if the oil is cold pressed.

It is also important that the carrier oil that you are going to use is fresh as well as pure. In order to keep the oil's freshness, make sure that you keep it away from the heat. It is even advisable to store your carrier oil away from a place where it can be hit directly by the light.

The shelf life of the carrier oil is also an important factor to consider whenever you are going to use this oil. You must also make sure that your carrier oil still has not exceeded its shelf life. (We have listed in the previous chapter how long some carrier oils usually last.) Again, make sure that your oil is still fresh, or at least its shelf life still has not ended. Some experts suggest that you add about 10 percent jojoba oil to your carrier oil—regardless what kind of carrier oil it is—for you to be able to prolong its shelf life. Jojoba oil, as well as other Vitamin E oil, will act as an antioxidant to your mixture, which in turn will extend the shelf life of your oil.

We have also mentioned in the previous chapter that the mixture should be composed mostly of carrier oils. Basically, essential oils should just make up the 2 percent of the mixture. (You do not need to exceed by at least one percent; 2 percent is *enough*.) Always keep in mind that essential oils are highly concentrated and it will be harmful for the skin if you apply it undiluted. So make sure that you only apply enough essential oils onto your skin.

If you want to achieve just 1 percent dilution, then add only 6 drops of essential oils to an ounce of carrier oils. If you want 2 percent dilution, just add 12 drops of essential oils to an ounce of carrier oils.

More importantly, you only have to make enough mixture, depending on how long you will use it. For instance, if you are just going to use it once or twice, then it is better if you will make a small blend, which is just enough for that use. Do not make too much; it is better that you use fresh blends rather than those that have already been stored for so long.

Conclusion

Thank you again for purchasing this book!

I hope this book was able to inform you more about what carrier oils are and what they can do for our body. Moreover, I also hope that this book was able to help you know where as well as how to use carrier oils.

The next step is to keep at least a bottle of carrier oil at your own home so that you will be able to use it next time.

Finally, if you enjoyed this book, please take the time to share your thoughts and post a review on Amazon. We do our best to reach out to readers and provide the best value we can. Your positive review will help us achieve that. It'd be greatly appreciated!

Thank you and good luck!

Check Out My Other Books

Below you'll find some of my other popular books that are popular on Amazon and Kindle as well. Simply click on the links below to check them out. Alternatively, you can visit my author page on Amazon to see other work done by me.

Coconut Oil for Easy Weight Loss: A Step by Step Guide for Using Virgin Coconut Oil for Quick and Easy Weight Loss

http://www.amazon.com/Coconut-Oil-Easy-Weight-Loss-ebook/dp/B00JG8H8DE

Superfoods that Kickstart Your Weight Loss Learn How to Use 30 Superfoods to Boost Weight Loss, Immunity and to Live a Healthier Lifestyle

http://www.amazon.com/Superfoods-that-Kickstart-Your-Weight-ebook/dp/B00JNAPM9M

Carrier Oils for Beginners: Discover the Characteristics and Beauty and Health Benefits of Carrier Oils For mixing Aromatherapy Essential Oils

http://www.amazon.com/Carrier-Oils-Beginners-Characteristics-Aromatherapy-ebook/dp/B00K88GI2S

Natural Homemade Cleaning Recipes For Beginners: Essential Oil Recipes For Household Cleaning, Laundry & Toxic Free Living

http://www.amazon.com/Natural-Homemade-Cleaning-Recipes-Beginners-ebook/dp/B00K87UBQI

The Best Secrets of Natural Remedies: The Ultimate Guide to Natural Remedies to Prevent and Cure Illnesses, Cold and Flu for Your Family

http://www.amazon.com/Best-Secrets-Natural-Remedies-Illnesses-ebook/dp/B00JNDCOCM

The Hypothyroidism Handbook:An Everyday Guide to Natural Solutions of living with Hypothyroidism including increased energy, lasting weight loss, and general well-being

http://www.amazon.com/Hypothyroidism-Handbook-Solutions-including-increased-ebook/dp/B00JNIGIV0

The Hyperthyroidism Handbook: An Everyday Guide to Natural Solutions of Living with Hyperthyroidism including Weight Gain, Increased Energy and General Well-being

http://www.amazon.com/Hyperthyroidism-Handbook-Solutions-including-Hypothyroidism-ebook/dp/B00JOHU5SM

Essential Oils & Weight Loss for Beginners: Ultimate Guide to Losing Weight, Increasing Energy, Balancing Metabolism & Appetite Using Essential Oils & Aromatherapy

http://www.amazon.com/Essential-Oils-Weight-Loss-Beginners-ebook/dp/B00JOFOWP6

Top Essential Oil Recipes: A Recipe Guide Of Natural, Non-Toxic Aromatherapy & Essential Oils for Healing Common Ailments, Beauty, Stress & Anxiety

http://www.amazon.com/Top-Essential-Oil-Recipes-Aromatherapy-ebook/dp/B00JY434E2

Soap Making For Beginners: A Guide to Making Natural Homemade Soaps from Scratch, Includes Recipes and Step by Step Processes for Making Soaps

http://www.amazon.com/Soap-Making-Beginners-Homemade-Processes-ebook/dp/B00JYKH75I

Body Butters For Beginners: Proven Secrets To Making All Natural Body Butters For Rejuvenating And Hydrating Your Skin

http://www.amazon.com/Body-Butters-Beginners-Rejuvenating-Hydrating-ebook/dp/B00K6LVV6A

Apple Cider Vinegar For Beginners: Proven Secrets Using Apple Cider Vinegar For Health, Weight Loss, and Skin Care

http://www.amazon.com/Apple-Cider-Vinegar-Beginners-Aromatherapy-ebook/dp/B00K6YY6HI

Homemade Body Scrubs & Masks For Beginners: 50 Proven All Natural, Easy Recipes For Body & Facial Masks To Exfoliate Nourish, & Care For Your Skin

http://www.amazon.com/Homemade-Body-Scrubs-Masks-Beginners-ebook/dp/B00K79D4SY

Essential Oils Box Set #1: Essential Oils & Weight Loss For Beginners (Ultimate Guide to Losing Weight, Increasing Energy, Balancing Metabolism & Appetite Using Essential Oils & Aromatherapy) + Top Essential Oil Recipes (A Recipe Guide of Natural, Non-Toxic Aromatherapy & Essential Oils for Healing Common Ailments, Beauty, Stress & Anxiety)

http://www.amazon.com/ESSENTIAL-OILS-BOX-SET-Aromatherapy-ebook/dp/B00K7Q8HRK

Essential Oils Box Set #2: Essential Oils & Weight Loss For Beginners (Ultimate Guide to Losing Weight, Increasing Energy, Balancing Metabolism & Appetite Using Essential Oils & Aromatherapy) + Top Essential Oil Recipes (A Recipe Guide of Natural, Non-Toxic Aromatherapy & Essential Oils for Healing Common Ailments, Beauty, Stress & Anxiety)

http://www.amazon.com/ESSENTIAL-OILS-BOX-SET-Aromatherapy-ebook/dp/B00K7Q8HRK

Box Set#3: Coconut Oil for Easy Weight Loss(A Step by Step Guide for Using Virgin Coconut Oil for Quick and Easy Weight Loss) + Apple Cider Vinegar(Proven Secrets Using Apple Cider Vinegar for Health, Weight Loss, and Skin Care)

http://www.amazon.com/Box-Set-Beginners-Aromatherapy-Essential-ebook/dp/B00K9TEGUW

Box Set #4: Body butters For Beginners(Proven Secrets To Making All Natural Body Butters For Rejuvenating And Hydrating Your Skin) & Top Essential Oil Recipes: A Recipe Guide Of Natural, Non-Toxic Aromatherapy & Essential Oils for Healing Common Ailments, Beauty, Stress & Anxiety

http://www.amazon.com/Box-Set-Butters-Beginners-Essential-ebook/dp/B00KA02F4Y

Box Set #5: Soap Making For Beginners(A Guide to Making Natural Homemade Soaps from Scratch, Includes Recipes and Step by Step Processes for Making Soaps) + Homemade Body Scrubs & Masks For Beginners(50 Proven All Natural, Easy Recipes For Body Scrub & Facial Masks To Efoliate, Nourish, & Care For Your Skin)

http://www.amazon.com/Box-Set-Beginners-Homemade-Recipes-ebook/dp/B00K9U3I2I

Box Set #6: Body Butters for Beginners (Proven Secrets To Making All Natural Body Butters For Rejuvenating And Hydrating Your Skin) +Homemade Body Scrubs & Masks For Beginners(50 Proven All Natural, Easy Recipes For Body Scrub & Facial Masks To Exfoliate, Nourish, & Care For Your Skin)

http://www.amazon.com/Box-Set-Beginners-Exfoliating-Moisturizing-ebook/dp/B00K9U3Y4O

Box Set #7: TOP ESSENTIAL OILS(A Recipe Guide Of Natural, Non-Toxic Aromatherapy & Essential Oils For Healing, Common Ailments, Beauty, Stress & Anxiety) & THE BEST SECRETS OF NATURAL REMEDIES(The Ultimate Guide to Natural Remedies to Prevent and Cure Illnesses, Cold and Flu for Your Family)

http://www.amazon.com/BOX-SET-Essential-Recipes-Remedies-ebook/dp/B00K9WPMQG

Box Set #8: NATURAL HOMEMADE CLEANING RECIPES FOR BEGINNERS (Essential Oil Recipes for Household Cleaning, Laundry & Toxic Free Living) + TOP ESSENTIAL OILS(A Recipe Guide Of Natural, Non-Toxic Aromatherapy & Essential Oils For Healing, Common Ailments, Beauty, Stress & Anxiety)

http://www.amazon.com/BOX-SET-Beginners-Essential-Aromatherapy-ebook/dp/B00KAMNGBS

Box Set #9: Essential Oils & Weight Loss for Beginners (Ultimate Guide to Losing Weight, Increasing Energy, Balancing Metabolism & Appetite Using Essential Oils & Aromatherapy) + Carrier Oils for Beginners (Discover the Characteristics and Beauty and Health Benefits of Carrier Oils for Mixing Aromatherapy Essential Oils) http://www.amazon.com/BOX-SET-Essential-Beginners-Aromatherapy-ebook/dp/B00KAODL6Q

BOX SET #10: THE HYPERTHYROIDISM HANDBOOK (An Everyday Guide to Natural Solutions of Living with Hyperthyroidism including Weight Gain, Increased Energy and General Well-being) + THE HYPOTHYROIDISM HANDBOOK (Everyday Guide to Natural Solutions of Living With Hypothyroidism Including Increased Energy, Lasting Weight Loss, and General Well-Being)

http://www.amazon.com/BOX-SET-10-Hyperthyroidism-Hypothyroidism-ebook/dp/B00KAKMSBY

BOX SET #11: CARRIER OILS FOR BEGINNERS (Discover the Characteristics and Beauty and Health Benefits of Carrier Oils for Mixing Aromatherapy Essential Oils) + Essential Oils & Aromatherapy for Beginners (Secrets to Beauty, Health and Weight Loss Using Proven Essential Oil and Aromatherapy Recipes

http://www.amazon.com/BOX-SET-Beginners-Essential-Aromatherapy-ebook/dp/B00KAONEQ8

BOX SET 12: ESSENTIAL OILS & WEIGHT LOSS FOR BEGINNERS: (Ultimate Guide to Losing Weight, Increasing Energy, Balancing Metabolism & Appetite Using Essential Oils & Aromatherapy) + TOP ESSENTIAL OIL RECIPES (A Recipe Guide of Natural, Non-Toxic Aromatherapy & Essential Oils for Healing Common Ailments, Beauty, Stress & Anxiety) + CARRIER OILS FOR BEGINNERS (Discover the Characteristics & Beauty & Health Benefits of Carrier Oils for Mixing Aromatherapy Essential Oils) + ESSENTIAL OILS & AROMATHERAPY FOR BEGINNERS (Secrets to Beauty & weight Loss Using Proven Essential Oil & Aromatherapy Recipes) + NATURAL HOMEMADE CLEANING RECIPES FOR BEGINNERS (Essential Oil

Recipes for Household Cleaning, Laundry & Toxic Free Living)

http://www.amazon.com/BOX-SET-12-Essential-Aromatherapy-ebook/dp/B00KCBCHE4

BOX SET #13: SUPERFOODS THAT KICKSTART YOUR WEIGHT LOSS (Learn How to Use 30 Superfoods to Boost Weight Loss, Immunity and to Live a Healthier Lifestyle) + ESSENTIAL OILS & AROMATHERAPY FOR BEGINNERS (Secrets to Beauty, Health and Weight Loss Using Proven Essential Oil and Aromatherapy Recipes) + BODY BUTTERS FOR BEGINNERS (Proven Secrets To Making All Natural Body Butters For Rejuvenating And Hydrating Your Skin) + SOAP MAKING FOR BEGINNERS (A Guide to Making Natural Homemade Soaps from Scratch, Includes Recipes and Step by Step Processes for Making Soaps) + HOMEMADE BODY SCRUBS FOR BEGINNERS (50 Proven All Natural, Easy Recipes For Body Scrub & Facial Masks To Exfoliate, Nourish, & Care For Your Skin)

http://www.amazon.com/BOX-SET-Superfoods-Kickstart-Aromatherapy-ebook/dp/B00KC8G6DK/

BOX SET 14: Essential Oils & Weight Loss for Beginners (Ultimate Guide to Losing Weight, Increasing Energy, Balancing Metabolism & Appetite Using Essential Oils & Aromatherapy) + Apple Cider Vinegar for Beginners (Proven Secrets Using Apple Cider Vinegar for Health, Weight Loss, and Skin Care) + Body Butters For Beginners (Proven Secrets To Making All Natural Body Butters For Rejuvenating And Hydrating Your Skin)
+ Homemade Body Scrubs & Masks for Beginners (50 Proven All Natural, Easy Recipes for Body Scrub & Facial Masks to Exfoliate, Nourish, & Care for Your Skin) + Coconut Oil for Easy Weight Loss (A Step by Step Guide for Using Virgin Coconut Oil for Quick and Easy Weight Loss)

http://www.amazon.com/BOX-SET-Essential-Beginners-Aromatherapy-ebook/dp/B00KEDO68U

If the links do not work, for whatever reason, you can simply search for these titles on the Amazon website to find them.

www.ingramcontent.com/pod-product-compliance
Lightning Source LLC
Chambersburg PA
CBHW060224290526
45789CB00003B/1396